HERBAL FIRST AID

NATURAL MEDICINE

by Andrew Chevallier

BA(Hons) MNIMH

Published by
Amberwood Publishing Ltd
Mulberry Court, Stour Road, Christchurch, Dorset BH23 1PS
Tel: 0202 474445

'To my Father'

ISBN 0-9517723-5-X

Illustrations by Tony Weare

Typeset and designed by
Word Perfect, Christchurch, Dorset.

Printed in Great Britain

CONTENTS

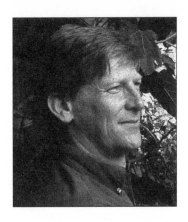

Andrew Chevallier

Andrew Chevallier is an experienced medical herbalist with a busy practice in Stoke Newington, North London, and in a hospital based complementary health clinic close by in Shoreditch.

He is a member of the National Institute of Medical Herbalists and currently its Vice-President and Director of Education. He is a council member of the Natural Medicines Society and of the Council for Complementary and Alternative Medicine.

He has made regular appearances talking about herbal medicine on radio and television and each summer leads herbal recognition walks throughout London.

Foreword

Dr Andrew Dunford
MB BS MRCGP DRCOG MNIMH

Andrew Chevallier has succeeded in distilling into this tiny book the precious essential oils from many thousands of years of folklore from all corners of the earth. Trial and error, or some deep and as-yet ill-understood intuition, have gradually led those members of any society entrusted with the business of healing to the use of simple and effective remedies from their immediate environment. How amazing, for instance, that comfrey should now be shown to contain the chemical necessary to increase the rate of healing of bone and cartilage, and that hundreds of years ago this property was so well known in England that the plant's common name was knit-bone. How sad too, that modern bureaucracy should try to prevent us using such a valuable plant through some theoretical risk of some of its ingredients, when the modern alternatives to some of its uses include the corticosteroids – with all their serious side-effects.

Indeed it may be the gradual realisation of the inherent untrustworthiness of so many modern drugs that will lead people to try out the remedies contained in this book. There is a happiness that comes from making a tea out of the leaves of a lime tree, or using the deliciously-perfumed oil of the thyme bush that we grow in the window-box, which is missing when it comes to scored white pills, or garishly-coloured capsules covered in indecipherable medical hieroglyphics. A patient of mine with AIDS used to tell me how he would smile when it came to swigging his twice daily dose of the herbal medicine tincture – not only was it without side-effect, but it made him feel that Nature herself was willing him to get better, indeed that Nature was smiling on him. And the more we try to understand about what goes on inside as the body tries to heal itself the less we really know. But what is becoming more and more obvious is that how you feel about your illness – and the treatments you are using – has an enormous effect on the eventual outcome.

In its U-turn on natural systems of medicine, the British Medical

Association points to the increasing interest seen among younger doctors in these forms of therapy. In one recent study of eighty-six GP trainees, eighteen already used at least one alternative method, while seventy wanted further training in one or more techniques.

The same BMA report describes herbalism as 'systems of treatment in which various parts of different plants are used to restore function and to treat symptoms'. Here lies the focus of this book — trying to explain in simple and understandable terms how our local plants help to strengthen the body's own deep desire to restore its normal healthy functioning, while at the same time accepting that we all live in the real world where babies yell with toothache, and that this doesn't have some deeply meaningful usefulness for their later psychological development — it merely drives everyone in the household into a frenzy of searching for a quick and effective symptomatic remedy. And if the remedy is also cheap and safe, then so much the better. I can just picture the harassed mum snatching this little book off the kitchen table, and see the relief on her face as she busies herself making up an infusion of camomile or elderflower tea, then mixing some of her slippery elm powder into a paste and applying it — gently but firmly — to the offending gums. And as if by magic, she feels she's doing something so natural and safe, and as old as the world itself, that her anger subsides, the baby feels its miseries have been properly noted, and order is restored once again to the household.

At least that is the idea. One of the bits of fun from this book will be to test out what works for whom, and the freedom to experiment safely with the healing powers supplied in such abundance for us by Nature herself.

1 | Introduction

This is a small book that could have been much larger! Knowledge of herbs is growing all the time but the needs of a 'first aid' book are for it to be small and easy to read, and this book has been written with these needs in mind.

As a practical book the whys and wherefores of plant medicine have been left out. What is left in is straightforward advice for simple herbal first aid treatment.

Through this book you will be able to experience first hand the effectiveness of herbal medicine – its strengths and subtleties – and should quickly be able to treat minor injuries and illnesses with confidence.

This book is not an alternative to conventional first aid books – these explain *emergency* first aid measures. It offers first aid advice for non-urgent day to day health problems, known as 'self-limiting' in the medical world. You should find the herbs to be gentle, effective and safe. If you notice no signs of improvement or you begin to get worse, in spite of taking herbal medicines, you should seek professional advice from your GP or qualified medical herbalist.

2 | How to use this book

1) Look up the ailment you need (e.g. Coughs) in the A–Z of Ailments. Read the *whole* section for the ailment. At the top of each section is a list of herbs that can be readily used to treat or alleviate the ailment.

2) Look up the herb or herbs you are going to use (e.g. Thyme) in the A–Z of Herbs, so that you can be clear about how and when to use them.

3) If you are not familiar with how to use or make up a herb, look up the How to Use Herbs section which will tell you exactly how to make up a herb tea, a poultice and so on.

4) Use the herb as suggested, taking into account the age of the person taking the herb (if a child see 'Children' page 11).

5) Often you will find that herbal medicines work quickly, but you should allow time for healing to take place as well. Herbal medicines work with your body's natural healing powers and so will not always bring instant results.

Also use this book to build up your own HERBAL FIRST AID BOX for home and travel. See page 14.

Lastly, if you really want to be a resource for your family and friends take a first aid course with the St. John's Ambulance Brigade or the Red Cross. And read more about herbal medicine – see the Booklist on page 47.

3 | Cautions

All the herbal medicines in this book are extremely safe, but they are still medicines! Treat them with respect. The biggest problem with self-treatment lies in not getting professional advice when it is needed. So use your common sense and:-

If in doubt seek urgent professional advice from a GP, or medical herbalist, or casualty department.

Do not put off seeking this treatment if you or someone you are looking after is clearly unwell. This includes:-

possibly broken or fractured bone
severe blow to the head
constant head pain
severe pain of any kind
significant difficulty in breathing
fever of 39°C/102°F or more
noticeable change in behaviour, including feeding patterns of babies

If you are taking long term medication from your GP or hospital it is wise to check first – with a medical herbalist or GP – that herbal medicines are safe for you to take, though it is *very* unusual for there to be a problem in this way.

4 | Pregnancy

All the herbs in the book *except for Feverfew and Sage* are safe to take during pregnancy. Some are especially helpful – Camomile, for example, is often helpful in morning sickness. During pregnancy it is wise to take medicines only when they are really needed - this is also true for herbal medicines.

5 | Children

Children need smaller amounts of herbs than adults - check the Dosage section if giving herbs to children. *Except for Feverfew,* all the herbs in this book are safe for children when given at the right dosage.

Note: Peppermint and Sage are not suitable for children under 4 years. See also 'Children's Ailments', page 30.

6 | How to use herbs

Once you have decided what herb to use you must choose how to use it. Teas (or infusions), decoctions and poultices all have to be made up, while tinctures, tablets and ointments or creams are ready to use. Essential oils usually need to be diluted in Almond or Sunflower oil.

Leaves and flowers, fresh or dried, should be chopped up and made as teas. Roots and barks need to be made as decoctions.

Teas
Use 1 small handful of fresh herb or 1 heaped tsp of dried herb to a cup of boiling water, or use 25g (1oz) to ½l (1 pint) of boiling water to make 3 cups at a time. Make in a teapot or put a saucer on top of the cup, stir, leave to stand for 5-10 minutes. Strain, drink while hot. Can be kept for up to 24 hours in a fridge.

Decoctions
EITHER use 25g (1oz) of root or bark to ¾l (1½pints) of boiling water and simmer for 15 minutes in an open saucepan – this will make 3 cups: OR grind until a powder and use 1 tsp to a cup of boiling water, stir, cover and leave to stand for 5-10 minutes. In both cases strain. Can be kept for up to 2 days in a fridge.

Poultices
Are most easily made using powdered herbs, especially Slippery Elm or Comfrey Root. Mix with enough hot water or Marigold tea to make a thick paste. Put this on to lint or muslin (or a sterile dressing on an open wound) fold over, and apply firmly to inflamed and sore areas. Fresh or dried chopped herbs e.g. Comfrey Leaf, can also be used scald leaves with hot water, drain and wrap in lint.

Compresses
Soak a clean flannel or cloth (or lint) in a herb tea and place it on to sore or painful skin.

7 | Dosage

All the dosages given throughout the book are, unless it says otherwise, the standard adult dose. This is:-
  1 cup of herb tea 3-4 times a day, or
  1 cup of decoction 2-3 times a day, or
  1 tsp (= 5ml) of tincture 2 times a day with water

Take tablets according to the instructions on the label.

Essential oils are normally diluted so that the maximum amount of essential oil is 5% = 5 drops of essential oil to 1 tsp (= 5ml) of Almond or Sunflower oil. In a bath add 5 drops in total. Essential oils should not be taken internally without professional guidance.

As one gets older so the capacity of the body to break down and remove medicines decreases. If you are 70 or over, take up to 2-3 cups of herb tea a day, or 1-2 cups of herbal decoction, or 1-2 tsps (= 5ml) of tincture, as appropriate.

Children under 1 year should have $\frac{1}{10}$th of the adult dosage; or if the mother is breastfeeding she can take the standard adult dose. Between 1-6 years take $\frac{1}{3}$rd of the adult dose; between 6-12 years $\frac{1}{2}$ the adult dose. Use essential oils on children under 4 years only in a very dilute form – 1-2 drops of essential oil at the most to each tbsp (= 20 ml) of Almond oil. From 6-12 use half the adult dose.

8 | The herbal first aid box

The 10 herbs listed below are those most helpful in first aid problems and minor infections. These 10 – when used together with the bandages, sticking plasters, thermometer etc. of a normal first aid kit – make a very effective herbal first aid box.

Aloe vera gel
Arnica ointment
Comfrey ointment
Echinacea tablets (or tincture)
Garlic capsules (or fresh)
Lavender oil
Marigold ointment and tincture
Slippery Elm tablets (or powder)
Thyme oil (and herb)
Ti-tree oil

If you buy all these in small quantities you will have a compact and portable herbal first aid kit – quite small enough to take away on holiday and able to help with everything from sunburn to insect bites and stomach upsets!

9 | A-Z of herbs

LIST OF HERBS IN THE A-Z SECTION

Aloe vera
Arnica
Camomile
Comfrey
Cornsilk
Cramp Bark
Dandelion
Echinacea
Elderflower

Eyebright
Fennel
Feverfew
Garlic
Lavender
Limeflowers
Marigold
Meadowsweet
Nettle

Passiflora
Peppermint
Sage
Slippery Elm
Thyme
Ti-tree
Valerian

ALOE VERA ~

gel, compress

acne, bites & stings, burns, chilblains, cuts, itchiness, sunburn, wounds

Known as the 'First Aid Plant' in the USA Aloe vera is drying and protective for the skin, powerfully increasing the rate of healing of burns, wounds and skin problems. It is even used for radiation burns! Buy the gel, soak in cotton wool and dab directly on to the sore, spot or wound. Better to keep a plant and break off a leaf to release the gel when needed! (Use only the juice, not the yellow sap). Bandages soaked in the gel come off more easily when removed. A very useful remedy for many first aid situations.

ARNICA~

ointment, cream

back pain, bruises, joint pain, muscle aches, sprains

Caution: not to be used on open wounds or broken skin.

Arnica ointment, if applied straight after a blow or sprain, quickly reduces both pain and swelling, making it particularly useful for bruises. It is helpful in general muscle aches, drawing the circulation to the area and warming it. Some skins may be sensitive to it, so apply carefully the first time you use it.

CAMOMILE ~ *tea, tincture, compress, poultice, cream, essential oil*

allergies, asthma, children's ailments – colic constipation sleep teething; diarrhoea, hay fever, hiccup, indigestion acidity & vomiting; itchiness, period pains, poor sleep, sore breasts, sore eyes, shock, stomach aches & pains, sunburn, wind

Camomile is extremely useful in many digestive ailments e.g. acid indigestion, while its simple relaxing properties make it helpful in shock, tension and anxiety.

For babies and children it will help in bedwetting, irritability and overtiredness. Camomile is used for nightmares and night terrors and encourages a sound night's sleep. Itchy and allergic skin conditions, including eczema, can be eased by Camomile tea – as a lotion or add it to a bath. For sore eyes soak the tea in cotton wool and apply to lids, or use a warm tea bag as a compress. Inhale the tea or essential oil in hayfever.

A poultice of Camomile flowers soothes sore breasts – apply warm to the breast and hold in place until cooled.

Make Camomile tea in a closed container (a cup with a saucer on top will do). For short term use, use 1 heaped tsp of dried flowers or 2 teabags per cup up to 5 times a day.

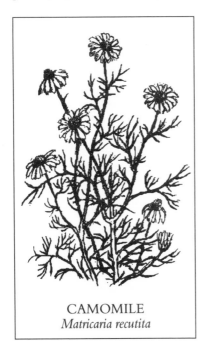

CAMOMILE
Matricaria recutita

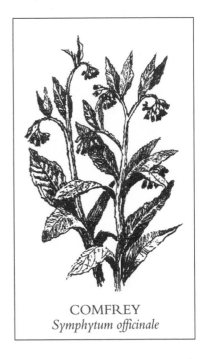

COMFREY
Symphytum officinale

COMFREY ~   *ointment, cream, poultice*
acne & boils, back pain, bruises, cuts grazes & wounds; fractures & sprains,
itchiness, joint pain, scars

THE herbal remedy for broken bones, sprains and fractures – it is essential
in the herbal first aid box. Rub the ointment in to the damaged area
(where the skin is broken use Marigold) as quickly as you can, the sooner
applied the more swelling and pain will be avoided. Comfrey also helps
to heal scars – old and new. For acne and boils add 5 drops of Ti-tree oil
to each 10g of ointment – mix it well in and put on the affected skin.

CORNSILK ~   *tea, tincture*
cystitis, water retention

Cornsilk is the silk-like fronds found wrapped inside a corn on the cob.
Dry and keep them in an airtight container until needed. Being antiseptic
and soothing it is helpful in bladder and urinary infections. As it increases
urine flow it is helpful in water retention and bloating, especially if pre-
menstrual. Cornsilk is very light so use 1 heaped tbsp to a cup, and take
up to 4 cups a day.

CRAMP BARK ~   *tincture, tablets, decoction*
anxiety & tension, asthma, back pain, constipation, hiccups, joint pain,
muscle aches & cramps, period cramps, stomach aches and pains

As the list suggests Cramp Bark will bring relief to colicky and cramping
problems, relaxing overtense muscles, and it is therefore an important
pain reliever. Cramp Bark goes well with Camomile and Valerian where
stress is the cause of the muscle tension, perhaps in conditions like
'irritable bowel' and mild asthma. It will help in constipation only where
this is due to overtightness of the bowel. For short term use you can take
1 tsp (= 5ml) of tincture up to 5 times a day, for example, to relieve period
pains.

DANDELION ~   *decoction, tincture*
acne, allergies, constipation – adults and children, hangovers, hay fever,
water retention, warts

By supporting and cleansing the liver Dandelion Root improves the
removal of waste products and is an ideal herb for toxic conditions such
as hangovers. Useful too taken internally in skin conditions like acne, and

allergies like hay fever, but only if taken for some weeks. Dandelion Root is a gentle laxative and is quite suitable for constipation in children.

To treat warts find a Dandelion plant and apply the white juice that is released when the leaf or stem is broken, twice a day for a few weeks. Dandelion Leaf is a good herb for water retention, as its common name of Piss-a-bed suggests!

Root – take 1-2 cups a day of the decoction or 1 tsp twice a day of the tincture. Instant dandelion 'coffee' is very much a second best! Leaf – take 1-2 cups a day of the tea.

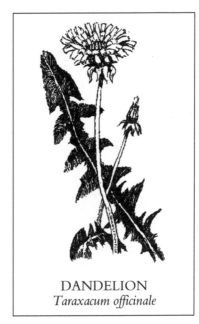

DANDELION
Taraxacum officinale

ECHINACEA ~
tincture, tablets, decoction

acne & boils, asthma, bites & stings, bronchitis, catarrh & sinuses, children's infections, colds & flus, cold sores, cuts and grazes, cystitis, digestive infections, earache, mouth ulcers, shingles, sore throats, thrush, warts

Good for all infections Echinacea is a highly useful plant, essential in any herbal first aid box. Take it to raise the body's resistance to infection or to speed recovery. Use with other herbs according to the nature of the problem e.g. Sage and Thyme for sore throat, Elderflower for colds and flu. For cold sores, shingles and skin infections take Echinacea internally and try applying the tincture neat externally as a strong natural antiseptic. Echinacea can safely be taken with antibiotics and helps to reduce their side-effects, especially thrush. Maximum dosage of the tincture is 1 tsp (= 5ml) 2 times a day. Do not overuse Echinacea – take it only when you really need it.

ELDERFLOWER ~
tea, lotion/eyebath, tincture

bronchitis, catarrh & sinus problems, children's ailments – infections & teething; colds & flus, coughs, earache, eye problems, hay fever, nosebleeds, sore throats

Elderflower tea brings warmth and relief to those suffering from colds, flus and chesty conditions. Safe and effective for children it checks fevers and reduces catarrh. Add honey, lemon and a pinch of Ginger or Cayenne for greater effect. Strain Elderflower tea carefully and use lukewarm in an eyebath for conjunctivitis, sticky eyes and similar problems. Or apply the tea soaked in cotton wool as a compress. Elderflower may give relief to hayfever and sinus problems but the effect may only be lasting after some weeks' treatment. Take up to 6 cups of tea a day for 2-4 days for colds and flus; babies ¼ dose, children ½ dose.

EYEBRIGHT ~ *tea, tincture, eyebath*
allergies & hay fever, catarrh & sinus problems, colds & flus, earache, eye problems, nosebleeds

As its name suggests Eyebright is useful for many eye problems. For sore, inflamed and infected eyes and lids, and especially if there is a discharge, make a normal strength tea and strain carefully. Allow to cool to body temperature, pour into an eyebath and bathe eyes well up to 3 times a day. Alternatively add 3-4 drops of tincture to an eyebath of warm spring water. Eyebright is good for the mucus membranes of the nose and sinuses helping to control the symptoms of hay fever. Mix it with Elderflower for best results in hay fever and catarrhal states. Eyebright is drying so do not take more than 2-3 cups of tea a day, tincture up to ½ tsp 2 times a day.

FENNEL ~ *tea, seeds*
children's ailments – colic; eye problems, hangovers, hiccup, indigestion acidity & vomiting; travel sickness, wind

A remedy for weak and sensitive digestions Fennel relieves wind, nausea and bloating. As a children's herb it will also help in griping, colic and vomiting. Fennel taken whilst breastfeeding increases breast milk production, and reduces colic and wind in the feeding baby. The tea well strained and applied in an eyebath is beneficial for sore, tired and inflamed eyes – or use a tea bag as a compress over closed eyes.

FEVERFEW ~ *fresh leaf, tablets (fresh leaf much better)*
bites & stings, headache, joint pain, migraine, period pains

Caution – not to be taken during pregnancy, when breastfeeding or given to children under 12 yrs. Some people are sensitive to Feverfew and it can cause mouth ulcers – try a small piece of leaf first before taking the normal dose.

A strong herb to be used carefully, Feverfew can relieve a variety of painful conditions. It is best known for its ability to relieve headaches and migraines – eat 1-2 leaves in a piece of bread. Feverfew can also help with arthritic and period pains. In all cases take Feverfew before the pains have built up and become severe. Feverfew makes a good insect repellent and the tea applied to insect bites and stings will reduce pain and swelling. Take the fresh leaf up to a maximum of 3 times a day only when you need to; follow instructions on label for tablets.

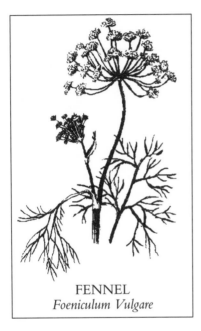

FENNEL
Foeniculum Vulgare

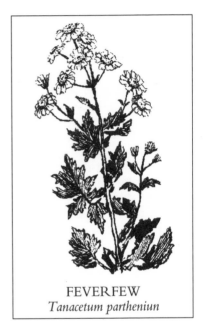

FEVERFEW
Tanacetum partheniun

GARLIC ~   *fresh, capsules, tablets*
acne, athlete's foot, asthma, bites & stings, bronchitis, catarrh & sinus problems, colds & flus, cold sores, coughs, digestive infections, earache, gum problems, mouth ulcers, shingles, sore throat, thrush, warts, wind

Garlic is one of nature's wonders. A natural antibiotic it can be taken in all types of infection, particularly those affecting the nose, throat and chest. Best to take a raw clove of Garlic chopped or crushed in with food 2-3 times a day for infections (or follow the recipe below). Tablets and capsules are fine too. Mouth ulcers, infected gums and sore throats will all respond to a clove of Garlic sucked and held in the cheek – for the brave or Garlic lover only!

Garlic is strongly anti-fungal and can help with thrush and athlete's foot. Like Echinacea it can be taken with antibiotics to reduce their side-effects. For ear infections put 2-4 drops of Garlic oil – from a garlic capsule – on a cotton wool plug and put it carefully in to the ear oily end first.

An excellent mixture for colds and flus:-

Add 1 chopped clove of Garlic, ½ tsp fresh or dried Ginger, fresh Lemon juice, and 1 tsp of Honey - mix together, cover with hot water and drink it all down. Take up to 3 times a day.

For long term use as a food supplement take 1 clove a day.

LAVENDER ~   *essential oil, tea*

allergies, anxiety & tension, burns, bites & stings, cold sores, cuts and grazes, earache, headaches, hiccup, itchiness, joint pains, muscle aches, period pains, poor sleep, shingles, sunburn, teething

Lavender is a gentle pain reliever and should be part of every first aid kit. Lavender oil (unlike most essential oils) can be applied neat – rub a few drops into the temples for headache and migraine, or put it directly onto insect bites and stings. It will also act as a mild insect repellent. For larger areas dilute the oil – 5 drops to 1 tsp (= 5ml) of Almond or Sunflower oil – and rub firmly into painful areas, e.g. over the womb for period pains. Lavender oil helps to heal burns – gently spread neat oil onto burnt and sunburnt skin. 5 drops in a bath will help relieve tension and encourage a good night's sleep.

Lavender tea has much the same properties as the oil but is much less concentrated and so can be taken internally – for anxiety, tension and low spirits, and for difficulty in sleeping. Take 1 cup up to 2 times a day.

LIMEFLOWERS ~   *tea*

anxiety & tension, catarrh & sinus problems, children's ailments – infections & sleep; colds & flus, headaches, migraines, PMT, poor sleep, shock

Limeflowers is the right herb if you are starting to feel stressed. Completely safe for adults and children it relieves headaches and calms the mind. Difficulty in sleeping, nervousness, and panic all respond well. Limeflower tea is very useful in colds and flu where headache and sinus congestion are the main problem. It is also very helpful for nervous palpitations. It tastes delicious – drink up to 5 cups of tea a day

MARIGOLD (CALENDULA) ~

tea, tincture, ointment, cream, compress

acne, allergies, athlete's foot, bites & stings, burns, chilblains, children's ailments – cradlecap, nappy rash; cold sores, cuts grazes & wounds, digestive infections, eye problems, infected gums, itchiness, nosebleeds, rashes, sore nipples, splinters, styes, sunburn, thrush, warts, wind, wounds

Marigold is the antiseptic and healing herb for red, sore and angry skin problems. Apply the ointment or cream and Marigold's healing and anti-inflammatory effect will quickly start to work. To cleanse an infected cut or graze rinse well with water (use a shower head at moderate pressure) then dab on neat or diluted tincture soaked in cotton wool or lint this will sting but is powerfully antiseptic. For young children dilute 1 part tincture to 4 parts water. Washing a cut in carefully strained Marigold tea is also very effective.

Dab neat tincture or ointment on acne spots. For infected or deep splinters, boils, whitlows and similar problems mix Marigold tincture with Slippery Elm (see page 24). Marigold is a very useful remedy for fungal problems – put ointment or powder on athlete's foot, ringworm etc. Use Marigold tea (strained) as a douche or sitz bath in thrush and vaginal soreness.

Taken internally Marigold tea eases heartburn, acidity and upset digestion. Marigold is very safe for children – use the ointment for nappy rash and inflamed and itchy skin, and the tea as a rinse for cradle cap.

The flowers are very bulky so use 1 heaped dessertspoonful per cup, and take up to 4 cups a day. For a lotion or compress use enough boiling water to just cover the flowers. The tincture, which is normally 90% alcohol, is an excellent anti-septic but is not really suitable to take internally. Ointment and cream can be applied as often as wanted.

MEADOWSWEET ~

tea, tincture, tablet

back pain, cystitis, diarrhoea – adults and children, heavy periods, indigestion & acidity, joint pain, muscle aches

Meadowsweet is helpful for upset stomachs and acid indigestion as well as providing relief in mild diarrhoea. It is often used for arthritic aches and pains and combines well with Devil's Claw tablets. Combine it with Nettle to reduce bleeding in heavy periods. Can be mixed with Cornsilk for mild cystitis. For short term use take up to 5 cups a day.

NETTLE ~

tea

acne & boils, allergies, cystitis, hayfever, heavy periods, nosebleeds, rashes, wounds

Despite its sting Nettle is a very useful and much underrated herb! It is high in iron and speeds up the rate of clotting of wounds, both factors making it helpful for loss of blood. Nettle can often bring relief in allergic reactions such as nettle rash and hay fever (use with Elderflower). In all of these situations try drinking 4-5 cups of Nettle tea a day for a few days and then reduce to 2-3 cups a day. Remember that you can use the fresh plant as a tea – pick in an unpolluted area and use gloves!

PASSION FLOWER/PASSIFLORA ~   *tea, tablet, tincture*
anxiety & tension, asthma, earache, headache, migraine, period pains, PMT, poor sleep children and adults, shock, toothache

Passiflora is mildly sedative and relieves many types of aches and pains. It is calming in anxiety and panic. It mixes well with Valerian in overactivity. Together, these two herbs are good for shock and that shaken up feeling after an accident. Passiflora encourages a sound night's sleep, and soothes ear- and tooth-ache. For short term use take up to 4 cups of tea a day.

PEPPERMINT ~   *tea, tincture, essential oil*
colds & flus, diarrhoea, hangovers, headache, hiccup, indigestion, itchiness, travel sickness, wind

Caution – not advisable for children under 4 years
Peppermint brings relief to indigestion, nausea and wind and is useful in a wide range of digestive ailments, especially when combined with Camomile. Mix it with Elderflower to make an effective remedy for colds and flus. It will ease headaches, especially if combined with Limeflowers. Apply Peppermint tea as a lotion to soothe and cool itchy skin – or put it in a bath. The oil is much stronger and should only be used diluted – mix 2-3 drops of the oil in 1 tsp of Marigold ointment to soothe itchy skin and itchy scabs.

SAGE ~   *tea, tincture*
bites & stings, catarrh, colds & flus, diarrhoea, gum problems, mouth ulcers, sore throats

Caution – not advisable during pregnancy or when breastfeeding. Not suitable for children under 4 years.
Use Sage tea as a gargle or mouthwash for quick results in relieving sore throats, mouth ulcers, and sore gums. Its astringent and healing action also makes it useful in diarrhoea. Sage benefits almost all cold and catarrhal states and is a good digestive tonic. It will reduce excessive sweating and

hot flushing. Fresh crushed leaves rubbed on to insect bites or stings will help pain and swelling. For greater effectiveness try adding a pinch of Cayenne pepper to the tea when using it as a gargle! Sage is a strong tea so do not take more than 3 cups a day.

SLIPPERY ELM ~ *powder, tablets*
boils, bronchitis, children's ailments – colic constipation teething; constipation, coughs, diarrhoea, indigestion & acidity, rashes, splinters, toothache

A wonderful, soothing herb, Slippery Elm can produce dramatic results in acid indigestion, gastritis, gastro-enteritis, diarrhoea, constipation, bronchitis, and coughs. For all of these conditions use Slippery Elm 'food'– see below. A lost filling can be temporarily plugged with Slippery Elm. To make a very effective drawing poultice for boils, splinters and whitlows mix 1 tsp of Slippery Elm with sufficient Marigold tincture to make a thick paste. Put the paste carefully on to the infected area and bandage it in place (put olive oil on first if the area is hairy!). In most cases the splinter or pus will have been drawn within a few hours. Repeat if necessary.

Slippery Elm 'food' – mix 1 heaped tsp of powder to a paste with cold water, then pour on ½l (1 pint) of boiling water and stir. Add cinnamon, nutmeg, lemon rind or honey to flavour and drink whilst warm. Take 1-4 times a day. It will help in all the internal ailments listed above. Tablets are not as effective but are still useful.

THYME ~ *tea, tincture, essential oil*
asthma, athlete's foot, back pain, bronchitis, catarrh & sinuses, children's infections, colds & flus, coughs, hay fever, joint pain, muscle aches, sore throats, thrush, warts

Use Thyme tea for all kinds of infections of the air passages – from the ear to the lungs. It has a strong antiseptic and calming effect making it valuable in earache, sinusitis, chest infections and the like. In these ailments Thyme combines well with Garlic and Echinacea. Use this combination also for thrush and other fungal problems.

Thyme syrup is a pleasant remedy for children's coughs or simply sweeten Thyme tea with honey. Burn Thyme oil over an essential oil burner to cleanse a room and speed the recovery of the patient – especially in chesty conditions. Inhale Thyme tea (or a few drops of Thyme oil in a basin of hot water) for relief of catarrh and sinusitis. You can also dilute Thyme oil 5 drops to 1 tsp (= 5ml) of warm Almond oil and rub firmly into the chest and back in all chesty conditions.

TI-TREE ~
essential oil

acne & boils, athlete's foot, colds & flus, cold sores, infected – bites & stings, rashes, cuts and wounds; shingles, thrush, warts

Caution – do not apply ti-tree oil neat on young children

Ti-tree oil is a potent yet gentle antiseptic. Apply it neat to small areas such as an acne spot, or around a nail, but if the area is larger than the size of a 50p piece it is advisable to try it diluted first – use about 10 drops to 1 tsp (= 5ml) of Almond oil or Marigold ointment. Even diluted Ti-tree oil can sting so be careful putting it on sensitive areas - and keep it well away from the eyes. You can also apply the oil diluted in a lotion such as Aloe vera gel – 2-3 drops per tsp of gel, and shake well – to prevent infection taking place on grazes, wounds, and so on. Ti-tree is one of the most useful herbal first aid remedies and should be in every first aid kit.

VALERIAN ~
tincture, tablet

anxiety & tension, asthma, back pain, headaches, migraine, palpitations, period pains, PMT, poor sleep – adults and children, shock

Valerian is a relaxing and calming herb that has no connection at all with 'Valium'. Though it is clearly not addictive, people do have very different levels of sensitivity to it – so the first time you try Valerian take a small dose e.g. ½ tsp of tincture or 1 tablet. If this is not strong enough take more as required until you find the right dose for yourself. Valerian eases tension and panic and relieves muscle pains and cramps. It can be helpful on its own for period pains but is better mixed with Cramp Bark. It is safe to give to children but use it as a last resort – try Camomile or Limeflowers first if your child cannot sleep or is overactive. For adults it is one of the most helpful remedies for insomnia.

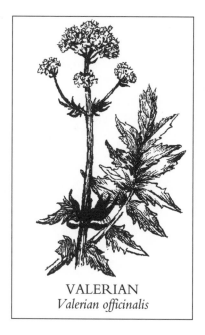

VALERIAN
Valerian officinalis

10 | Kitchen medicines

Even if you do not have the herbs recommended in the A–Z section you may have useful herbal medicines in your kitchen without realising it. Remember that many cooking herbs have a medicinal use too – these can be used dried or straight from the garden.

BEETROOT – rich in iron; good for anaemia; inhale juice through the nose to cleanse catarrh – see 'Catarrh & Sinuses'!

CABBAGE – scald or iron a large leaf and apply hot, as a poultice in swollen and inflamed conditions.

CAYENNE – good for poor circulation and chilblains; add a pinch to gargles – do not make too strong!

CINNAMON – good for colds as a tea.

CLOVES – anaesthetic and antiseptic – chew a clove for toothache.

CUCUMBER – cooling, put slices on hot, sore eyes etc.

DRIED FRUIT – mild laxative for constipation.

GINGER – an excellent herb for colds, indigestion and sickness. Use in cooking or make a tea.

HONEY – antiseptic, containing natural antibiotics. Apply to wounds. Useful as soothing sweetener in teas for coughs and colds.

LEMON – antiseptic and cleansing. Helps the body cope with infection.

LEMON BALM – a relaxing and pleasant flavoured herb tea. It is calming for anxiety, and settles nervous indigestion. The herb and the essential oil are strongly antiseptic to cold sores.

MINT – garden mint can be used instead of Peppermint

PARSLEY – useful in cystitis, and arthritis; very rich in vitamins and minerals, especially vitamin C and iron.

ONIONS – similar to garlic only milder in effect.

ROSEMARY – a warming and cheering herb tea that raises the spirits when depressed. Add 5 drops of essential oil to a bath, for its invigorating effect in the morning.

11 | A–Z of ailments

ACIDITY - see Indigestion

ACNE & BOILS – aloe vera, comfrey, dandelion root, echinacea, garlic, marigold, nettle, slippery elm, ti-tree

Acne spots develop where the oil glands of the skin have become blocked, so caring for the health of the skin is as important as treating individual spots. For 'first aid' treatment of acne spots apply Aloe gel, Comfrey or Marigold ointment, either on its own or mixed with Ti-tree oil or Echinacea. Or dab neat Marigold tincture onto the spots. Lemon juice and Garlic can also be useful.

Boils are a sign of being run down and unlike acne they go deep into the skin. If you get them often consult your GP or medical herbalist. Treatment is the same as for acne but use the Slippery elm drawing poultice described on page 24, and take Echinacea and Garlic internally. Adjusting your diet cutting down on 'junk' food and dairy produce, and eating more vegetables and fruit will help too.

ALLERGIES & HAY FEVER – camomile, dandelion root, elderflower, eyebright, lavender, marigold, nettle, thyme

In an allergic reaction cells leak out into the surrounding area causing swelling, itchiness and redness. It can be a minor irritation or an emergency – if in doubt seek urgent medical advice.

Red, itchy or swollen skin which comes up after contact with chemicals, plants, jewellery or from some other cause will be soothed by Marigold or Camomile, or better still both together. Soak a flannel or clean cloth in the tea and hold in place. Adding Camomile or Lavender oils or applying either oil neat will also be helpful. Drink large amounts of Nettle tea and at the same time apply it as a lotion. Chickweed cream, or juice squeezed from the fresh plant, will relieve itchiness.

For hay fever take frequent cups of Elderflower and Nettle tea (mixed in equal parts). Inhaling Camomile or Thyme oil can help to stop sneezing and irritation. These oils are strong so use in this way for no more than a day or two at a time.

ANXIETY & TENSION – camomile, cramp bark, lavender, limeflowers, passiflora, valerian

Symptoms of stress and panic are familiar to everyone – tense neck muscles, tight breathing, feeling irritable or panicky and so on. Herbs can bring significant relief. Valerian is especially valuable helping one to relax and unwind even when very anxious. Take Limeflower tea for panic and palpitations. Camomile is the best herb for anxiety in children. Cramp bark as its name suggests relaxes muscle tension.

All these herbs will be more effective if you take other steps to relieve stress – do some form of relaxing exercise or slow deep breathing for example, and avoid drinking too much tea or coffee.

ASTHMA – camomile, cramp bark, echinacea, garlic, passiflora, thyme, valerian

Caution – do not try to use herbs instead of medication from your GP or hospital. See a medical herbalist if you wish to do this. Asthma can be a life threatening condition DO NOT DELAY seeking proper emergency treatment.

Tight-chestedness and mild asthma can be relieved with a mixture of Thyme, Camomile and either Cramp bark or Valerian – this will help to open up the airways and encourage relaxed breathing. Drink lots of this as a tea; it can also be inhaled under a towel. Thyme is specific for asthma and is very suitable for children. Thyme, Echinacea and Garlic are extremely useful if the tight-chestedness is due to a chest infection. 2 drops each of Camomile and Thyme essential oil in 1 tsp (= 5ml) of almond oil rubbed on to the chest and upper back is well worth trying. Apply 2-3 times a day for a few days.

ATHLETE'S FOOT – garlic, marigold, thyme, ti-tree

Not strictly a first aid problem, athlete's foot can flare up and be a real nuisance. Mix Thyme or Ti-tree oil in Marigold ointment – 5 drops to 1 tsp (= 5ml), and apply 2-3 times a day. Alternatively if the area is small put on neat Ti-tree oil. Avoid wearing socks and shoes made of synthetic materials, and dry your feet carefully after bathing – a nonperfumed talc may help. Treat fungal problems affecting the skin and nails as described above.

BACK PAIN – arnica, comfrey, cramp bark, lavender, meadowsweet, thyme, valerian

For back pain caused by accidents rub Arnica or Comfrey ointment into the painful area. You can add Lavender oil too 5 drops to 1 tsp (= 5ml) of ointment. If heat helps the problem, a thyme compress or hot bath with lots of Thyme tea strained into it can bring significant relief. Or add 4 drops each of Thyme and Lavender oil and stir well into the bathwater. Use a hot water bottle!

If the pain is due to muscle tension it will respond well to Cramp bark or Valerian. Sometimes you can get astonishing results in this way. If the pain is due to arthritis, Meadowsweet or Feverfew may ease it.

BITES & STINGS – aloe vera, echinacea, feverfew, garlic, lavender, marigold, sage, ti-tree

Aloe vera gel and Marigold ointment soothe and heal bites and stings, and reduce the chances of infection. Neat Lavender oil or fresh Sage leaves can also be rubbed on to bites and stings. A vinegar compress will help to neutralise wasp stings; baking soda dissolved in water and applied as a compress helps bee stings. Apply Marigold ointment or Lavender oil immediately afterwards. Use Echinacea, Garlic or Ti-tree if the bite becomes infected.

Insects can be repelled by using Lavender oil or Feverfew rubbed onto exposed areas. If desperate, eating plenty of Garlic, or cutting it and rubbing into the skin will put off most insects but may discourage humans as well!

BOILS – see Acne

BRONCHITIS – echinacea, elderflower, garlic, slippery elm, thyme

Garlic is excellent for bronchitis and deep chesty coughs eat plenty crushed fresh in to your food or take capsules. Echinacea tablets will be helpful too to fight the infection. Thyme and Elderflower make a very good tea that eases breathing and coughing. Thyme oil diluted in almond oil – 5 drops to 1 tsp (= 5ml) and warmed to body temperature makes a good chest rub. Bronchitis thrives on cold, damp and polluted air – keep warm and perhaps use an ioniser! Burn Thyme oil in your bedroom.

BRUISES – arnica, comfrey

Bruises will heal rapidly and effectively with frequent applications of Comfrey ointment or poultices. Arnica is also extremely helpful. Apply as soon as possible after an injury (arnica to unbroken skin only) and you will help to keep the bruised area to a minimum. If the skin is broken, see 'Cuts'.

BURNS – aloe vera, lavender, marigold

Firstly, burns can be a medical emergency – if the burn is severe or deep even over a small area, get immediate medical assistance. Secondly, burns need cold water – wherever the burn either immerse it directly in cool, clean water or soak clean sheet and wrap carefully around the burnt area. Keep cold for up to 3 hours – not only does this relieve pain but it reduces the damage to the burnt area. Once cooled apply lots of Aloe vera gel. Thirdly, if the burn is severe but covers a small area only, bandage with lint (soaked in aloe vera if possible) and give the patient a drink of water with ½tsp of Valerian tincture or 4 drops of the Bach Flower Rescue Remedy added. Both will help to ease the shock. If the burn is suitable for home treatment and you do not have Aloe vera gel, apply Marigold ointment or neat Lavender oil – both are very healing and Lavender will help to relieve pain. If nothing else is available use honey – it is sterile and contains natural antibiotic substances. For minor scalds cucumber slices are cooling and soothing.

CATARRH & SINUS PROBLEMS – echinacea, elderflower, eyebright, garlic, limeflowers, sage, thyme

Mix Elderflower, Limeflower and Thyme tea (add a pinch of cayenne pepper for greater effect!) to reduce catarrh production and soothe and relieve many catarrhal problems you can drink lots of it, up to 6 cups a day for a week if necessary. Echinacea and Garlic are very helpful too, cleansing and improving the resistance of the nasal membranes to infection. Thyme and Peppermint tea can be inhaled from a basin – put a cloth over your head and breathe in the steam. Lastly, try sniffing salt water or beetroot juice through your nose. Sniff up through a straw! It sounds unpleasant but can bring a lot of relief. Also, cut your intake of dairy produce and sugar. These foods are 'fuel on the fire' of catarrhal problems.

CHILBLAINS – aloe vera, marigold

Take a piece of fresh ginger root and squeeze the juice over unopened chilblains. You can do the same with lemon juice. Marigold ointment and Aloe vera gel will help to heal open sores and reduce itchiness. Taking Garlic regularly will improve circulation in the long term.

CHILDREN'S AILMENTS – Colic, Constipation, Diarrhoea, Cradlecap, Infections, Nappy rash, Sleeplessness, Teething

Herbal medicine is well suited to children. Camomile, Elderflowers, Fennel, Limeflowers, Marigold, Nettle and Thyme are particularly safe for children and can be given to babies and infants with confidence.

Dosage is important – check the section on page 13. Getting your child to take any form of medicine can be a struggle and herbal medicine is not an exception. The earlier you start giving herbs to children the better – before they are conditioned to say 'it tastes horrible and yukky!'

Teas and tinctures may be mixed with honey, or diluted apple juice, although it is better to give them unsweetened especially to young children. Tablets can be crushed and mixed with honey etc. A bath can be an easy way to give herbs to babies and young children – especially for itchiness and overtiredness. If you are breastfeeding take the adult dose of the appropriate herb for your child and he or she will get it in the right proportion within your breastmilk.

COLIC
Camomile and Fennel are well known for relieving colic and wind. They are best taken as unsweetened teas. Camomile tea strained into a bath can also help. If breastfeeding adjusting your diet may help! Also, feed your baby in as peaceful a situation as possible. When weaning, Slippery elm powder can be made up as a gruel and is very soothing for sensitive young digestions. It is also very nutritious.

CONSTIPATION
Camomile tea and Slippery elm 'food' (see pages 16 and 24) are again the herbs of choice here. Eating wholemeal bread or porridge oats will usually help – providing sufficient roughage; also eat figs, dates and raisins. Dandelion root is a mild laxative and is helpful for children prone to constipation.

DIARRHOEA
Children with severe diarrhoea are at risk from dehydrating. Make sure that they have lots to drink. Diluted fresh lemon juice with honey or sugar is best. Meadowsweet tea is often effective in relieving diarrhoea in children; you can also try Camomile. If the diarrhoea is uncontrolled consult your GP or medical herbalist.

CRADLECAP
Apply olive or wheatgerm oil to the scalp and let it soak in well. Marigold ointment is also useful. Apply either 1-2 times a day.

INFECTIONS

Children often run high fevers – sometimes when they are not ill in any other way - so it is important not to worry unduly if your child has a fever. Provided that the temperature is not over 39°C/102°F your child is unlikely to need the support of your GP or herbalist. Give regular cups of Elderflower, Limeflower or Meadowsweet tea. These herbs all help to keep a fever under control. Echinacea and Thyme are suitable for young children suffering from infections and will improve their resistance and rate of recovery. Thyme and Elderflower together are very good for chest infections. Putting your child in a cool bath will help to control a fever but if she or he starts to feel cold wrap them up well.

NAPPY RASH

Aloe vera gel, and Comfrey or Marigold ointment (rather than a cream) will help with this common problem. Dry the affected skin as much as possible – you can even use a hairdryer on the 'cool' setting – and allow your child time without a nappy on as much as possible. Sometimes nappy rash can be complicated by thrush – if this could be the case try adding 1 drop of Ti-tree oil to 1 tsp of Marigold ointment and apply at each change.

SLEEPLESSNESS/IRRITABILITY/OVERACTIVITY

Herbs are ideally suited for soothing a child who will not or cannot relax. Camomile is the first herb of choice – as a tea or in the bath – but if not strong enough try Limeflowers. Both of these can be given to children frequently if need be. In emergencies you can give children Passiflora or Valerian both most easily taken as tablets or tinctures. These herbs will usually get even the most excited child off to sleep but they should not be used regularly.

TEETHING

The grumpiness and discomfort that teething causes is not always easy to prevent! Camomile or elderflower tea will help to relieve fractiousness and irritability. Slippery elm powder made into a paste and rubbed in to the gums can be very soothing. Or rub diluted lavender oil, 2-3 drops to 1 tsp (= 5ml), externally on the cheeks over the site of the teething.

COLDS & FLUS – echinacea, elderflowers, garlic, limeflowers, peppermint, sage, thyme, ti-tree

The simplest cold and flu mix is elderflowers and peppermint. This makes a relaxing and refreshing tea that really does take the edge off some of the symptoms. Add Limeflowers if headache is a problem. Use Sage for sore throats, and with Peppermint for gastric symptoms. For more serious colds and flu take Echinacea, Garlic or Thyme as well. All of these will encourage a speedier recovery. Thyme and Ti-tree oils can be used in an essential oil burner, or put a few drops on the pillow or a handkerchief. Lastly take the Garlic and Ginger recipe on page 21 2-3 times a day.

For flu and in fevers resist eating unless you have an appetite. Concentrate on drinking fresh fruit juices and plenty of herb teas and water. Lemon and lime are particularly good. The suggestions above are often helpful but remember that in the young and old, flu can sometimes be a dangerous condition. If the fever is above 39°C/102°F or if you feel very unwell, seek professional advice.

COLD SORES – echinacea, garlic, lavender, marigold, ti-tree

Where possible prevention of cold sores is better than cure. If you are prone to these taking Echinacea and Garlic at times when they are likely to occur can be effective. Once you know that a cold sore is on its way, try gently rubbing fresh Garlic, ginger or lemon balm on to the area. Once the sore has opened you can still put these on but Marigold ointment may be the most helpful – perhaps, mixed with a little Ti-tree or lavender oil, 2 drops to 1 tsp (= 5ml).

CONSTIPATION – cramp bark, dandelion, slippery elm

Take Slippery elm tablets or linseed (1tbsp with cereal each morning) on a daily basis helps to help regulate bowel habits. Dandelion root is a mild laxative that should be tried first, along with dietary changes (see below), before thinking about taking a strong laxative like senna. Senna should be used only for those situations where nothing else has worked. If you have to take senna or some other strong laxative regularly see a medical herbalist. If constipation is a frequent problem then first look to your diet – eat foods like raw carrots, apples, porridge oats and wholemeal bread as well as dried fruit such as figs and prunes. Drink plenty of water. Do regular, pleasurable exercise..

COUGHS – echinacea, elderflower, garlic, slippery elm, thyme

Stubborn dry coughs will respond well to Elderflower and Thyme tea and Slippery Elm 'food' (see page 24). Together they will soothe the irritated airways and encourage the coughing up of sticky thick phlegm.

For coughs where a lot of phlegm is being produced take 2-3 cloves of

Garlic a day – preferably crush fresh cloves into your food although the capsules will do. For chest infections take Echinacea as well. A chest rub with 5 drops of Thyme oil to 1 tsp (= 5ml) of almond oil warmed and massaged over the chest will be pleasant and effective. There are a number of herbal cough mixtures available – Vegetable Cough Remover is particularly good.

CRAMPS – see Muscle Aches

CUTS, GRAZES & WOUNDS – aloe vera, comfrey, echinacea, lavender, marigold, ti-tree

For all but serious wounds herbal first aid is safe and effective. It will promote healing and help to prevent scarring. The aim is to reduce bleeding, cleanse, relieve pain and heal! To stop or slow bleeding press firmly on the cut and maintain pressure for 1-2 minutes. Take Nettle tea to help stop bleeding. Cleanse using strong Marigold tea, or add 5 tsp of Marigold or Echinacea tincture to a cup of boiled water. Soak pieces of cotton wool and gently wash out grit, glass etc. until the wound is quite clean. Now put on Marigold or Comfrey ointment, or Aloe vera gel, and bandage or cover with a sticking plaster.

If a cut or wound becomes septic use 5 drops of Ti-tree oil mixed with a tsp of Marigold ointment and apply every 2-4 hours. You can use Lavender in place of ti-tree – it is not so antiseptic but will sting less and give more pain relief. If the cut is not large use the Slippery elm drawing poultice to draw out the infection. Mashed Garlic is also very effective for septic wounds – put in muslin and hold in place.

CYSTITIS – cornsilk, echinacea, nettle

Cystitis is infection of the bladder and urinary tubes. It can be mild with frequent urination and a burning pain or it can be acute, with fever, significant pain, blood in the urine and the danger of infection spreading up to the kidneys.

In the home, mild cases of cystitis can be treated by following a few simple rules: drink lots of water and herb teas especially Cornsilk (though Nettle will help too); eat plenty of parsley and celery; drink diluted unsweetened cranberry juice if available; avoid tea, coffee, alcohol, orange juice and hot spices; and most important of all – keep warm and use a hot water bottle. You can use these suggestions in acute cystitis too but you should see a medical herbalist or GP as well. If symptoms are linked with sexual activity be fastidious about hygiene and empty bladder before and after penetration.

DIARRHOEA – camomile, echinacea, garlic, marigold, meadowsweet, peppermint, sage, slippery elm See also Children's Ailments

Diarrhoea can be a healing response by the body to eliminate toxins in the gut and it is better not to 'stop it in its tracks' unless you have to. (NB Children dehydrate very easily, see page 31). Drink large amounts of water or diluted lemon or carrot juice. Slippery elm food (page 24) is also important. For diarrhoea caused by gastro-enteritis, if your stomach will allow it, take Echinacea, Garlic or Marigold all of which will raise your resistance to the infection. You should take these as well, along with acidophilus capsules, if you have diarrhoea as a result of taking antibiotics. Meadowsweet, Peppermint and Sage will reduce the irritation of the gut that causes the diarrhoea, thus helping to keep the problem under control. If the diarrhoea is mainly a nervous 'irritable' type problem then Camomile and Meadowsweet are the herbs of choice.

EARACHE – echinacea, elderflower, eyebright, garlic, lavender, marigold, passiflora, thyme

Firstly treat any infection by enhancing the body's resistance to infection – take Echinacea and Garlic (Marigold will be useful too). Secondly use herbs that will help to reduce the amount of irritation and catarrh in the ear, nose and throat Elderflower and Thyme will reduce pressure and help to clear the passageways around the ear. Thirdly rub Lavender oil around the outside of the ear to help relieve pain. Passiflora can help to relieve pain.

Putting antiseptic oils into the affected ear can bring relief but never put anything into the ear if you think the eardrum may have burst – for example if there is a discharge from the ear. Put 2-3 drops of Garlic oil from a Garlic capsule on a cotton wool plug and gently insert it in to the ear; or do the same with Lavender oil. If the problem continues for more than a few days or is severely painful seek professional advice.

EYE PROBLEMS – camomile, elderflower, eyebright, fennel, marigold

Herbal first aid for common eye problems is often successful and if you follow the suggestions below you should get good results in all but stubborn cases.

Conjunctivitis or 'red-eye' – Make Eyebright tea at normal strength and filter carefully. When it reaches body temperature put in a clean eyebath and bathe affected eyes thoroughly for a couple of minutes. You can do this 3-4 times a day . A few grains of salt added to the eyebath will help too. Alternatively add 2-4 drops of Eyebright tincture to an eyebath of warm spring water. Elderflower tea made in the same way is also effective.

Strained and tired eyes – rest is obviously the best answer but also use a Camomile or Fennel teabag (from which you have just made a cup of tea)! Place the warm teabag over the closed eye and hold in place for a few minutes. Both are soothing and relaxing. A slice of cucumber on tired hot eyes is very refreshing.

Styes – being so close to the eyes styes can be difficult to treat. Either put Marigold ointment carefully on to the spot or soak warm Marigold tea in cotton wool and hold over the closed eye. Take Garlic or Echinacea if this is a recurrent problem.

'Things in the eye' – dust and insects in the eye should be washed out using Marigold or Eyebright tea. Though they may not manage to remove the object, they will reduce soreness and prevent inflammation.

FRACTURES, SPRAINS & BROKEN BONES –
arnica, comfrey

Comfrey is the herb for all damaged bones and ligaments. Apply Comfrey ointment over the whole area as soon as possible after the accident . A Comfrey poultice will be just as good. You can also take Comfrey leaf tea internally to further speed up the rate of healing – Comfrey's other name is Knitbone! If the skin has been broken put Marigold ointment on the wound and comfrey all around it. Arnica ointment may help to relieve pain and can also help to speed the rate of healing.

FUNGAL INFECTIONS – see Athlete's foot and Thrush

GRAZES – see Cuts

HANGOVERS – dandelion, fennel, peppermint

There are 3 immediate things you can do to help a hangover:1) drink lots of water or diluted fruit juice – especially lemon juice, 2) drink a cup or two of Dandelion root coffee (the roasted root tastes very good), 3) if you can manage it eat bananas and salads, especially watercress. All these will help to break down and flush out alcohol from your body, and to replace some of the lost vitamins and minerals. When you can manage it, eating foods high in B vitamins will be helpful e.g. wholemeal bread, wheatgerm, oats. Carrot and Beetroot juice are cleansing and nutritious.

For queasiness take Fennel, Ginger or Peppermint tea. A hangover is a sign that you have intoxicated or poisoned yourself – if you are getting hangovers more than once a month you should look to the cause.

HAY FEVER – see Allergies

HEADACHES & MIGRAINES – feverfew, lavender, limeflowers, peppermint, valerian

Headaches can develop for many reasons – anxiety, eye strain, and neck tension for example – so try to work out what is causing it. Limeflowers are soothing and relaxing for many types of headache and bring relief especially where tension is the main cause. Both Peppermint and Valerian go well with limeflowers – Peppermint where indigestion is also a problem, and Valerian where stress is the major cause. Where sinus congestion is the main problem Elderflower and Limeflowers together work very well, relieving aches and reducing catarrh.

Gently massaging your neck and scalp will often help to relieve a headache. Rub a few drops of Lavender oil onto your temples or the back of your neck. Feverfew is the best herb for migraines though the herbs suggested above will be helpful too. Try and take the Feverfew before the migraine has started.

HICCUPS – camomile, fennel, lavender, peppermint

Although drinking water from the wrong side of a glass may be as effective as any other treatment Camomile, Fennel and Peppermint have all helped to bring relief to hiccups at one time or another! Try it out! Diluted Lavender or Camomile oil massaged firmly over the belly area is helpful.

INDIGESTION, ACIDITY & VOMITING – camomile, fennel, meadowsweet, peppermint, slippery elm

Indigestion and acidity are probably treated better with herbal medicine than anything else and there is a wide range of herbs to choose from. Meadowsweet tea is specific for acid indigestion and will generally bring quick relief. It goes well mixed in equal parts with Camomile or Marigold, and these two teas are also effective in their own right, settling indigestion and nausea. Fennel is more helpful where wind is the major problem. Slippery elm 'food' can be invaluable taken regularly before meals, helping to protect and soothe the stomach from irritation. Use Peppermint for indigestion or wind, or add it to any of the other herbs to give a pleasant flavour. Camomile, Fennel and ginger teas all help to ease nausea and vomiting – use 1-2 slices of fresh ginger root per cup. If you get frequent digestive problems go and see a herbalist. He or she will not only give you suitable herbs but advise you about what to eat, and not to eat!

INFLUENZA – see Colds and Flu

INSOMNIA – see Poor Sleep

ITCHINESS & SKIN RASHES – aloe vera, camomile, comfrey, lavender, marigold, peppermint, See also Allergies

For very itchy skin try any of the herbs listed above that you have readily available. Camomile and Marigold teas are likely to be helpful, especially if mixed together and applied as a lotion. Marigold cream on its own or with 2-3 drops of Camomile, Lavender or Peppermint oil added per tsp (= 5ml) will also be effective. If the skin is weeping use Aloe vera gel. Chickweed cream if you can find it is extremely good, or gather the fresh plant and squeeze the juice directly on to itchy areas. If the problem persists see a medical herbalist.

JOINT PAIN & STIFFNESS – arnica, comfrey, cramp bark, feverfew, lavender, meadowsweet, nettle, thyme

For short term relief of joint pain and stiffness, first ask yourself if the joint is hot, and perhaps swollen, or whether it is cold. If hot a pack of frozen peas put on the joint will help to cool it and reduce the pain. Lavender oil diluted 10 drops to 1 tsp of almond oil (or better still St. John's Wort oil) and massaged in gently will bring relief. If cold, use heat – have a hot bath. Add strong Thyme tea, or 5 drops of rosemary oil, or ½kg/1lb of Epsom Salts to it and soak for 20-25 minutes. Or use a hot water bottle or a hot compress Comfrey or cabbage (see 'Kitchen medicines') will reduce the pain. You can also try rubbing in Arnica ointment.

Meadowsweet and Cramp bark, taken internally, can help to reduce pain whether the joint is hot or cold. Feverfew, again internally, is worth trying as a pain reliever if no other treatment has worked.

MENSTRUAL PROBLEMS – Heavy bleeding, Painful periods, Sore breasts, Pre-menstrual tension, Water retention

Herbal medicines have been used to treat menstrual problems for thousands of years. They work safely, in tune with the body's natural monthly changes. The recommendations provided here are for first aid treatment only. Consult a medical herbalist if you have ongoing difficulties with your cycle.

HEAVY MENSTRUAL BLEEDING – nettle

Nettle tea taken frequently when bleeding will help to reduce a heavy flow, and provide a good intake of iron at the same time. Other herbs can be helpful, such as raspberry leaf, shepherd's purse and yarrow. A good iron supplement is 'Floradix'.

PAINFUL PERIODS – camomile, cramp bark, lavender, passiflora, valerian

Herbs can bring quick relief to period pains and cramps. As its name suggests Cramp bark is very helpful for period cramps and pains – take 10ml of tincture up to 4 times a day. If emotional stress or tension is part of the problem take Valerian as well. Passiflora relieves pain but makes one sleepy. Massaging Camomile or Lavender oil (diluted 5 drops to 1 tsp of almond oil) over your womb and lower abdomen is often helpful, or add 5 drops of either oil to a bath.

PRE-MENSTRUAL TENSION – limeflowers, passiflora, valerian

First aid treatment for PMT will really only touch the surface of the problem. Herbal medicine can be extremely effective in preventing pre-menstrual symptoms but treatment normally takes a few months. In the short term you can try Valerian and Limeflowers together if the main problem is irritability and snappiness. For exhaustion and low spirits take rosemary tea, or put 5 drops of rosemary essential oil in a morning bath. For difficulty in sleeping take Passiflora. Avoid tea and coffee, and try to exercise regularly.

SORE BREASTS – camomile, marigold

For sore breasts make a Camomile poultice – make a tea with 2 tbsp of flowers to 1 mug of boiling water and leave to stand for 10 mins. Soak this tea in a flannel or wrap in fine cloth like muslin, and hold gently in place on the sore areas. Keep in place until it has cooled. Reducing your caffeine intake may well be helpful. For sore nipples apply Marigold ointment regularly – if breastfeeding, wipe off the ointment before feeding as the child may be put off by the taste and smell.

WATER RETENTION – dandelion root or leaf, cornsilk

Cutting down on salt is a good starting point for this problem. Take Dandelion root (or better the leaf) or Cornsilk tea, both of which encourage the kidneys to remove more fluid from the body and act as diuretics. Again regular exercise helps.

MIGRAINE – see Headache

MUSCLE ACHES & CRAMPS – arnica, cramp bark, lavender, meadowsweet, thyme

A hot bath, perhaps with 4-5 drops of Lavender or Thyme oil , and a good night's sleep, will often be enough to ease tired and aching muscles. If the problem is more persistent then rub Arnica ointment firmly into tender areas – it will usually bring quick relief. Muscle aches due to a viral infection (as with flu) need Echinacea and Elderflower internally.

If the problem is mainly 'rheumatic' see 'joint pain', and take Meadowsweet tea. Lastly for all muscle cramps take Cramp bark tincture and if necessary rub it in to the affected area; taking magnesium and vitamin B complex may also be useful.

NOSE BLEEDS – eyebright, marigold, nettle

Pinching the nostrils gently and drinking a strong cup of Marigold or Nettle tea will stop a nosebleed in most cases. Use 2-3 tsp of herb to a cup and take a further cup if needed. Take Eyebright if the nosebleed starts because of excessive sneezing or nose-blowing. The old tradition of a cold key or ice cube on the back of the neck, whilst pinching the nostrils, often works – though I do not know why!

PERIOD PAINS – see Menstrual problems

POOR SLEEP – camomile, lavender, limeflowers, passiflora, valerian

Herbal medicine can be extremely helpful for insomnia and you run no risk of becoming addicted. Camomile is mild, and suitable as a relaxing night time drink, especially so if indigestion plays a part in the poor sleep.

Limeflowers is stronger – helping to calm anxiety and slow the pace of one's thoughts. Passiflora is definitely sedative and will often help one back to sound sleeping habits. Take it with Valerian if you are getting off to sleep without difficulty but wake in the early hours with your mind unable to 'switch off'. Also try a hop pillow. Put dried hops in a small pillow and go to sleep inhaling their aroma – a traditional and often effective remedy. Lastly, 5 drops of Lavender oil in a bath, and a few drops sprinkled on the pillow, can also ease you in to sleep.

PRE-MENSTRUAL TENSION – see Menstrual Problems

SHINGLES – echinacea, garlic, lavender, ti-tree

Shingles is a sign of nervous exhaustion. Eat plenty of oats, e.g. as porridge oats or oatcakes, as this is a 'food' for the nerves. To ease the pain and speed the healing of the blisters add 5 drops each of Lavender and Ti-tree oils to 1 tsp of almond or olive oil (St. John's Wort oil is better) and massage gently in. Take Echinacea and Garlic to improve resistance to the infection.

SHOCK – camomile, limeflowers, passiflora, valerian

Shocks can be eased by sipping Limeflower tea – use 2 tsp to a cup – and taking drops of the Bach Flower Rescue Remedy. Together they can have a very soothing effect. If anxiety is extreme take Valerian as well. For children Camomile tea may be enough on its own.

SINUSITIS – see Catarrh

SICKNESS – see Travel sickness

SKIN PROBLEMS – see Allergies, and Itchiness

SPRAINS – see Fractures

SORE BREASTS – see Menstrual problems

SORE THROATS – echinacea, elderflower, garlic, sage, thyme

Sage makes an excellent gargle for sore throats. Gargle with the tea or diluted tincture for a couple of minutes 2-5 times a day. Also mix it with other herbs to good effect e.g. Echinacea and Thyme. Swallow the gargle and get the benefit internally as well. For the brave there are 2 further suggestions – 1) add a pinch of cayenne pepper when making the tea to stimulate the body's resistance!, and 2) go to sleep with a clove of Garlic in your mouth – crush it between your teeth and keep in your cheek! Both of these are effective but slightly fierce ways of getting through a sore throat quickly.

Sore throats that turn into tonsillitis need lots of Garlic, Echinacea and Thyme. Sage and Elderflower will be useful too. In general avoid dairy produce and sugar rich foods. Drink fresh lemon juice and honey with warm water. See also 'Colds & Flus'.

SPLINTERS – marigold, slippery elm

Tweezers and a needle are the main needs, but herbal first aid can help in a surprising way. Deeply embedded splinters can be 'drawn out' using Slippery elm powder and Marigold tincture – see page 24. Apply the mixed paste over the splinter and keep firmly in place for at least 1-2 hours. Any pus is likely to have been drawn and the splinter should be much easier to remove. If not, repeat the process.

STINGS – see Bites

STOMACH ACHES & PAINS – camomile, cramp bark, garlic, marigold, peppermint

Pain is always a signal that something is wrong so do not just ignore stomach aches and pains, there are plenty of herbs that will bring relief. Herbal first aid centres on Camomile, Marigold and Peppermint. These 3 may be taken on their own or combined and will often soothe a troubled digestion. For colicky pains take Cramp bark and Camomile. Ginger tea – 1 level tsp of dried ginger root per cup – is very beneficial for stomach infections and goes well with Garlic.

SUNBURN – aloe vera, camomile, lavender, marigold

If the burnt area is small cover it with Marigold ointment or Aloe vera gel. Both will reduce the pain and stimulate the healing of the burn. If you have neither of these dab on cool Camomile tea which will also reduce the inflammation. Lavender is best used diluted – 3-5 drops per tsp (= 5ml) of ointment or gel. If the burnt area is large soak in a cool bath to which you have added lots of Marigold or Camomile tea or Aloe vera gel. See also 'Burns'.

THRUSH – echinacea, garlic, marigold, thyme, ti-tree

Vaginal thrush is increasingly common nowadays as it often develops as a side-effect of taking antibiotics, or in conjunction with spermicides. Drink 3-4 cups of Marigold tea a day, and use it locally as a douche or in a sitz bath. If this does not relieve soreness and itching use Ti-tree pessaries. These may sting to start with but are often very helpful. Also try putting live yoghurt into your vagina – it helps to soothe, and to counter the candida infection. You should also take Garlic and/or Echinacea tablets or tincture to help raise your immunity. For oral thrush all of the herbs listed above (except ti-tree) can be taken as mouthwashes. In general you should eat lots of Garlic and live yoghurt and avoid sugar, fermented foods, and alcohol.

TOOTHACHE, TEETH & GUM PROBLEMS – marigold, passiflora, sage, slippery elm

Cloves or clove oil are the best first aid remedy for toothache. Put one drop of the oil on the painful tooth or suck a clove next to it. Take Passiflora if the pain continues – it is very helpful in toothache but may make you sleepy. A lost filling can be plugged temporarily with chewing gum or slightly moistened Slippery elm powder. For sore and bleeding gums use Sage and/or Eyebright tea regularly as a mouthwash. For infected gums use either diluted Marigold tincture on cotton wool or suck a clove of Garlic! For mouth ulcers use Sage tea or tincture and dab neat on to ulcers. Also try dabbing neat clove oil onto them. Both will sting to start with.

TONSILLITIS – see Sore throats

TRAVEL SICKNESS & MORNING SICKNESS – camomile, fennel

A good strong cup of Camomile tea taken before a journey will reduce the chances of travel sickness – in children and adults. If you do not get on with Camomile, Fennel can be as effective. Research has shown that ginger tea – best to use a slice or two of fresh root per cup – is also very effective for sickness and nausea. All 3 herbs are well worth trying to relieve morning sickness. Where you are unable to make ginger tea, suck a piece of ginger root or crystallised ginger instead.

VOMITING – see Indigestion

WARTS – dandelion, garlic, marigold, thyme, ti-tree

Warts can be notoriously hard to get rid of, though they can also disappear overnight! The white juice from Dandelion leaves and stems put on twice daily for a few weeks will often remove warts. Also try Marigold ointment mixed with 4 drops of Ti-tree or Thyme oil per 5g/1 tsp of ointment. Garlic has a long term reputation for clearing warts - rub a cut clove onto the wart at least twice a day!

WATER RETENTION – see Menstrual Problems

WIND – camomile, echinacea, fennel, garlic, marigold, peppermint, sage

This can be a stubborn problem. Adjusting one's diet can make an immediate difference – dairy produce, wheat, fermented and sugary foods are often involved, and it may be worth trying to cut them out, in rotation for a week at a time.

Camomile, Fennel, and especially Peppermint are useful for windy digestions. Take them regularly. Sage tea is good for weak digestions helping to improve digestive function. Where wind is due to infection Garlic, Echinacea and Marigold will be beneficial.

WOUNDS – see Cuts

12 | Buying herbs and herbal medicines

Buying herbs that are of good quality is very important. If they have not been dried properly or they are old you can simply be throwing your money away. The best option is to grow as many herbs as you can in your own garden, or in some cases to pick them in the wild e.g. nettles.

Where this is not possible buy dried herbs from a local supplier who you know to be good. One way to judge whether the herbs are good quality is to look at the Marigold flowers stocked – if they are a beautiful deep orange colour they are fresh and in good condition, if they are yellowish or faded they are old and have probably been sitting on the shelf for too long!

Alternatively you can buy mail order. The 4 suppliers listed all take orders by letter or phone and provide good quality herbs, tinctures, powders, ointments and so on.

G. Baldwin & Co.
171/3 Walworth Road
London SE17 1RW
Tel: 071-703-5550

Napier & Sons
17 Bristo Place
Edinburgh EH1 1HA
Tel: 031-225-5542

Neal's Yard Remedies
4 Neal's Yard
Shorts Garden
London WC2H 9DP
Tel: 071-379-7222

Culpepper Ltd
Mail order
Hadstock Road
Linton
Cambridgeshire CB1 6NJ
Tel: 0223 891196
(17 branches throughout the UK)

Many herbal medicines can now be bought not only from health food shops but chemists. Herbal tablets are probably quite as effective as teas and they are very practical – easy to take and easy to carry about.

13 | Finding a herbalist

Looking under 'Herbalist' in the Yellow Pages may lead you to a good medical herbalist, but you can also write to the National Institute of Medical Herbalists, 9 Palace Gate, Exeter Devon EX1 1JA sending £1.50 for a list of members. All Members of the National Institute of Medical Herbalists have undertaken a 4 year course of study to qualify, and are governed by a professional code of ethics. They carry the initials MNIMH or FNIMH after their name. Members of the General Council and Register of Herbalists have not had such extensive training but are governed by a professional code of ethics. They carry the initials MH after their name.

14 | Booklist

There are so many books available on herbal medicine that it can get confusing. Here are some of better ones that go in to herbal medicine in more detail than this book can attempt to.

The New Holistic Herbal by David Hoffman (1990). Element. price £9.99.

Plant Medicine by Charlotte Mitchell (1991). Amberwood. Price £2.99

Herbal Medicine for Common Ailments by Anne McIntyre (1993). Gaia. Price £6.99.

The New Herbal ed. Richard Mabey (1988). £14.99

Out of the Earth by Simon Mills (1992). Viking. Price £25.

A Modern Herbal by Mrs. M. Grieve (1985). Cape. Price £25.

Green Pharmacy - A History of Herbal Medicine by Barbara Griggs (1981). Jill Norman & Hobhouse. Price £9.00.